Professional Standards for Occupational Therapy Practice

College of Occupational Therapists

Revised edition 2017

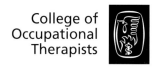

College of
Occupational
Therapists

This edition published in 2017
by the College of Occupational Therapists
106–114 Borough High Street
London SE1 1LB
www.cot.co.uk

Previous edition published in 2011. This edition supersedes all previous
editions.

Author: College of Occupational Therapists
Writer: Henny Pearmain
Category: Standards and strategy

Acknowledgements
With thanks to Members of the External Reference Group: Aisling Curran,
Lin Henry, Janet Kelly, Professor Pip Logan, Dr Jenny Preston, Dr Lee Price,
Manuela Schuette.

Other enquiries about this document should be addressed to the Assistant
Director of Professional Practice at the above address.

British Library Cataloguing in Publication Data
A catalogue record for this book is available from the British Library.

While every effort has been made to ensure accuracy, the College of
Occupational Therapists shall not be liable for any loss or damage either
directly or indirectly resulting from the use of this publication.

ISBN 978-1-905944-62-0

Typeset by Fish Books Ltd

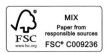

MIX
Paper from
responsible sources
FSC
www.fsc.org   FSC® C009236

Contents

Key terms

The College has selected or developed these definitions and explanations to help with the understanding of this document. If you are a member of the public and you need help understanding any element of this document, please ask your local occupational therapist.

Assessment	*A process of collecting and interpreting information about people's functions and environments, using observation, testing and measurement, in order to inform decision-making and to monitor change.* (Consensus definition from European Network of Occupational Therapy in Higher Education (ENOTHE) 2004)
Asset	*An 'asset' is defined as any factor or resource which enhances the ability of individuals, communities and populations to maintain and sustain health and well-being. These assets can operate at the level of the individual, family or community as protective and promoting factors to buffer against life's stresses.* (Hudson 2010)

Asset-based approach	An approach that values, utilises and builds upon the abilities, skills, knowledge and other resources of individuals, families, groups and communities. It aims to promote and strengthen the factors that support good health and wellbeing, enabling those individuals, groups and communities to gain more control over their lives and circumstances.
Autonomy	*The freedom to make choices based on consideration of internal and external circumstances and to act on those choices.* (Consensus definition from ENOTHE 2004)
Best interests	The best interests approach asks whether any proposed course of action is the best one for the service user, all things considered. As well as recognising the use of best interests decisions under the *Mental Capacity Act 2005* (Great Britain. Parliament 2005), the approach is extended within these standards to all service users. (Adapted from UKCEN (UK Clinical Ethics Network) 2011))
Care	'Care' is used in various ways in this document, talking about the care

	team, care documentation, etc. It is also used to encompass more than intervention, to capture the responsibility or attitudinal element, where the approach to our service users is one of care rather than neglect, as used in having a 'duty of care' or 'shared care' with another organisation. It also fits with the provision of both health and social care.
Carer	Someone who provides (or intends to provide), paid or unpaid, a substantial amount of care on a regular basis for someone of any age who is unwell, or who, for whatever reason, cannot care for themselves independently.
	(Adapted from Great Britain. Parliament 1995)
	This is sometimes divided into formal carers (care workers) who are paid to give care, and informal carers (often family) who are not paid to provide care.
Competence/ competency	*Competence is the acquisition of knowledge, skills and abilities at a level of expertise sufficient to be able to perform in an appropriate work setting.*
	(Harvey 2014)

Continuing professional development (CPD)	*CPD is a combination of approaches, ideas and techniques that will help you manage your own learning and growth.* (CIPD (Chartered Institute of Personnel and Development) 2016) *A range of learning activities through which health professionals maintain and develop throughout their career to ensure that they retain their capacity to practise safely, effectively and legally within their evolving scope of practice.* (Health and Care Professions Council (HCPC) 2012, p1)
Diverse settings	Working in settings or roles where occupational therapists traditionally have not worked.
Duty of care	A responsibility to act in a way that ensures that injury, loss or damage will not be carelessly or intentionally inflicted upon the individual or body to whom/which the duty is owed, as a result of the performance of those actions. A duty of care arises: ■ When there is a sufficiently close relationship between two parties (e.g. two individuals, or an individual and an organisation). Such a relationship exists

	between a service user and the member of occupational therapy personnel to whom s/he has been referred, while the episode of care is ongoing.
	■ Where it is foreseeable that the actions of one party may cause harm to the other.
	■ Where it is fair, just and reasonable in all the circumstances to impose such a duty.
	(See Caparo Industries plc v Dickman 1990)
Enablement	[The process of creating opportunities] *to participate in life's tasks and occupations irrespective of physical or mental impairment or environmental challenges.*
	(Christiansen and Townsend 2004, p276)
Generic role	A generic role may involve or practice combining tasks previously undertaken by different professions. This might be a part or all of a role. For example, providing management support across a range of professional groups, or carrying out a range of health checks within the community.

Professional Standards for Occupational Therapy Practice

Healthy occupations	Activities that encourage and develop health and wellbeing, or decrease the risk of injury or disease.
Intervention	*The process and skilled actions taken by occupational therapy practitioners ... to facilitate engagement in occupation.* (O'Brian et al 2012, p180)
Must	Where there is a legal requirement, an overriding principle or duty to act.
Occupation	*In occupational therapy, occupations refer to the everyday activities that people do as individuals, in families and with communities to occupy time and bring meaning and purpose to life. Occupations include things people need to, want to and are expected to do.* (World Federation of Occupational Therapists (WFOT) 2016)
Occupational performance	A person's ability to carry out the activities and roles that they need, or want, or are expected to do in their daily life.
Occupational therapy personnel	For the purpose of this document, this term includes occupational therapists, occupational therapists

	working in diverse settings or generic roles, occupational therapy students and support workers working with or for occupational therapists. It is also pertinent to occupational therapists who are managers, educators and researchers.
Outcome measure	*Outcome measurement can demonstrate the effectiveness of intervention for individual service users or population groups, guiding further decision-making and/or intervention. The use of outcome measures, especially standardised measures, allows occupational therapists to build up and use a body of evidence for occupational therapy.* (COT 2015b, p2)
Participation	*Participation is involvement in a life situation.* (World Health Organisation 2002, p10) *Participation can take on both objective (for example frequency) and subjective dimensions involving experiences of meaning, belonging, choice, control, and the feeling of participation.* (Eriksson et al 2007; Hemmingsson and Jonsson 2005 in Bonnard and Anaby 2016, p188)

Positive risk	Recognising and accepting, but managing, risk when there is a positive objective or outcome.
Practitioner	For the purposes of this document, see 'occupational therapy personnel'.
Reasonable	An objective standard. Something (e.g. an act or decision) is reasonable if the act or decision is one which a well-informed observer would also do or make.
Service user	For the purposes of this document the term 'service user' has a wide interpretation; relating to not just those in receipt of health and social care services but also to the population with whom you are working.
Should	Where the principle or duty may not apply in all circumstances, by contrast with a 'must' obligation.
Sustain/ sustainable	*Sustainable health care combines three key factors: quality patient care, fiscally responsible budgeting and minimizing environmental impact.* (Jameton and McGuire 2002)

Section One: Essential reading

1.1 Occupational therapy practitioners

Occupational therapy enables people to achieve health, wellbeing and life satisfaction through participation in occupation.
(College of Occupational Therapists 2004 definition, in World Federation of Occupational Therapists 2013, p48)

Occupational therapy practitioners are a highly skilled workforce operating across a wide range of settings, including health, social care, housing, education, research, employment, prisons and the third sector.

As an occupational therapist or a support worker, you are aware of your legal and professional obligations and how they impact upon your work. You always work within your competence and the remit of your job description and within the terms of your employment.

As an occupational therapist you are a qualified and competent professional. You are an autonomous practitioner and are personally accountable for what you do. You have a reasonable and demonstrable rationale for your practice (HCPC 2013, p5). You meet the requirements of the Health and Care Professions Council (HCPC) and are registered with them when practising within the United Kingdom.

1.2 The importance of occupation

Underpinning your practice is the belief that occupation and activity are fundamental to a person's health and wellbeing, within the context of their various environments. A person's ability to carry out the activities and roles that they need, want, or are expected to do in their daily life is seen as their occupational performance.

You understand how a person's health and wellbeing affects, and is affected by, their occupational performance and participation. Your professional practice is concerned with developing, maximising and/or maintaining service users' ability to engage in a range of occupations.

You enable a person, group or community to achieve their chosen goals through the modification of their desired or required occupations, learning new skills and approaches, adaptation of their environments, or a combination of these. You see activity in itself as an effective medium for remediation or an agent of change.

You take an asset-based approach, analysing and utilising the strengths of the individual, the environment, and the community in which a person lives and functions. You work with the person, their family and/or carers and their communities where appropriate, to identify solutions and enhance their ability to engage in the occupations they want, need, or are expected to do.

1.3 The role of the Health and Care Professions Council and the College of Occupational Therapists

The primary role of the Health and Care Professions Council (HCPC), as the regulating body, is the protection of the public. As an occupational therapist, you must be registered with the HCPC in order to practise within the United Kingdom and your professional practice must be carried out in accordance with their standards. If a formal complaint is made, or a concern is raised about a registrant's fitness to practise, the HCPC will take account of whether their own standards have been met (HCPC 2013, 2016).

The College of Occupational Therapists (COT) is the professional body and voluntary membership organisation for occupational therapists throughout the United Kingdom. It is a subsidiary of and trading name for the British Association of Occupational Therapists (BAOT), which also acts as a trade union. The College sets the professional and educational standards for the occupational therapy profession and represents the profession at national and international levels. A key function of the College is to support you, as members, informing and supporting you in your practice. It is not the role of the College to judge a practitioner's fitness to practise.

1.4 The professional standards

The *Professional standards for occupational therapy practice* are produced by the College, in consultation and collaboration with its members. They are developed in line with the Health and Care Professions Council (HCPC) standards in order to support you in meeting their requirements.

These standards should be read in conjunction with the *Code of ethics and professional conduct* (COT 2015a). Together they describe a level of practice and a set of professional values and behaviours that the College expects its members to abide by, and believes all occupational therapy practitioners should follow.

They are universal and applicable, with some interpretation, to all practitioners, irrespective of role or location. Whether an assistant, a new graduate or highly experienced; whether in a diverse setting or a generic role, you should be able to apply the underpinning principles of these standards to the work that you do.

In your practice you will need to use the knowledge and skills you have learned through education, experience and continuing professional development. You will also need to demonstrate behaviours that promote and protect the wellbeing of service users and their carers, the wider public, and the reputation of your employers and the profession. You also need to use national guidelines, research and evidence to underpin and inform your practice. Maintaining these standards will help you to:

■ be a safe and effective practitioner

■ provide a high-quality service

■ provide value for money

■ explain and promote the work that you do in the language of occupation

■ meet the registration requirements of the HCPC.

The *Professional standards* are very succinct in terms of describing what is expected of you. You are advised to read relevant COT guidance documents for further detail and explanation.

For students and educators these standards also complement the *College of Occupational Therapists' learning and development standards for pre-registration education* (COT 2014a) and *Entry level occupational therapy core knowledge and practice skills* (COT 2016), which describe the expected profile of an occupational therapy graduate. Both may be used to guide, develop and monitor the progress of students, graduates and returners to the profession.

These standards are an information resource to direct you and a means by which you can examine your practice. They may also be used as an aid to discussions in the workplace, whether with your colleagues, your manager or those you supervise. They may help to guide strategic decisions relating to occupational therapy and be used as a basis for dialogue and negotiation with commissioners, purchasers of services and in other business settings. You can use the standards to demonstrate the value and uniqueness of your professional contribution.

In any civil or criminal proceedings these standards may be admissible as evidence. They may be used as a measure of reasonable and/or acceptable practice in support of the complaint or the defence.

1.5 Terminology in these standards

Throughout these standards the term 'practitioner' has been used to identify you as the active individual, wherever you work and whatever your role. The term 'service user' has been used for those to whom you provide education, support, intervention or a service. This may sometimes be a group or a community. Although not always specified in the standards, the service user's carers and/or family should be actively involved where appropriate and with the agreement of the service user. The work that you do for and with service users has been termed 'care' and/or 'intervention'.

1.6 Monitoring and developing your practice and service

The Health and Care Professions Council (HCPC) requires you to 'be able to assure the quality of

[your] practice' recognising 'the need to monitor and evaluate the quality of practice and the value of contributing to the generation of data for quality assurance and improvement programmes' (HCPC 2013, section 12). You also have a responsibility to ensure that your service is optimised to meet identified need. Using these standards as a benchmark against which to scrutinise your practice and/or your service is one means of doing this. There are audit resources available on the College website to help you with this (www.cot.co.uk).

The results of monitoring and improving your practice should be included in your continuing professional development (CPD) portfolio, along with your other evidence of learning and development.

1.7 When local policy says different

You may find that occasionally local circumstances prevent you from meeting some part of the standards. In such a case, you need to be sure that you are meeting your legal responsibilities, your duty of care to service users and all HCPC requirements. If you are concerned that your local policy is causing you to fall short of your legal and professional duties, or that it puts the welfare of service users, yourself or your colleagues at risk, you must raise this with your employer. Keep a record of your concerns. You are advised to contact your local union representative and the College's Professional Practice Enquiries Service in such situations, as each may be able to advise you.

Section Two: Standard statements

■ These standards should be read in conjunction with the *Code of ethics and professional conduct* (COT 2015a).

■ Together they describe a level of practice and a set of professional values and behaviours that the College expects its members to abide by, and believes all occupational therapy practitioners should follow. They are applicable, with some interpretation, to all practitioners, irrespective of role or location.

■ Although not always specified in the standards, the service user's carers and/or family should be actively involved where appropriate and with the agreement of the service user.

1. **Underpinning your occupational therapy practice is an understanding of the relationship between occupation and health and wellbeing.**

    1.1 You understand how occupational performance and participation affects, and is affected by, a person's health and wellbeing.

    1.2 You understand the relationship between the person, their environment and their occupational performance and wellbeing.

1.3 You are able to explain and record your professional reasoning for anything you do for/with or in relation to service users.

1.4 Your practice is shaped or structured according to recognised theories, frameworks and concepts of occupational therapy.

1.5 You use national guidelines, research and other evidence to underpin and inform your practice.

1.6 In diverse settings or generic roles your practice still has an occupation focus.

2. Service users are at the centre of your practice.

2.1 You work in partnership with service users, being led and guided by their needs, choices and aspirations.

2.2 With the service user's agreement, you actively involve their carers and/or family in your practice as appropriate.

2.3 You seek to act in the best interests of service users to ensure their optimum health, wellbeing and safety.

2.4 You use the service user's preferred means of communication where possible, optimising their abilities to participate by any suitable means.

2.5 You uphold the service user's right to make choices over the care that they receive and the plans that they wish to make.

2.6 If a service user declines intervention or chooses to follow an alternative course of action, you do all you reasonably can to maintain his or her safety and wellbeing.

2.7 You assess and meet the needs of the carers where appropriate.

2.8 You work towards the inclusion and involvement of the service user in their own communities.

3. **Through review of documents, discussion and/or interview, you screen/triage the service user's occupational needs.**

3.1 You consider the occupational needs of the service user and the potential benefit of occupational therapy within the context of your service provision.

3.2 Where occupational needs are not present or could best be met through other service provision, you direct service users to alternative services, information and advice.

4. **Through interview, observation and/or specific assessment, you identify and evaluate the service user's occupational performance and participation needs.**

4.1 You use assessment techniques, tools and/or equipment that are relevant to occupation and appropriate to the service users and their circumstances.

4.2 Your analysis of the assessment outcomes shows how the service user's current situation or conditions affect their occupational performance and ability to participate.

4.3 If further assessments or investigations are indicated, you instigate these or refer to other services.

5. **You develop appropriate intervention plans, or recommendations, based upon the occupational performance needs, choices and aspirations of service users, as identified through your assessments.**

5.1 You work with service users in the planning process, agreeing their objectives and priorities for intervention.

5.2 You promote wellbeing, encourage healthy occupations and participation in life roles.

5.3 You act to reduce, delay or prevent future needs where possible.

5.4 You consider how the assets of the individual, their carers/family and their communities can be used to maximise their occupational performance.

5.5 You consider the impact of your intervention on the person, occupation and environment and how occupational performance and participation is affected.

5.6 You work with service users and relevant others to develop skills to manage their own occupational needs.

5.7 You agree and record timescales and/or review dates in your plans.

5.8 You review, amend and document your plans and interventions regularly in partnership with service users.

5.9 You work in collaboration with relevant others to inform your intervention.

6. **You evaluate the impact of the intervention that you have provided in terms of the service user's response and occupational outcomes.**

    6.1   You use outcome measures to monitor and review the ongoing effectiveness of your intervention.

    6.2   You include the views and experience of service users when evaluating the effectiveness of occupational therapy intervention.

    6.3   You take account of information gathered from relevant others.

    6.4   Where necessary you modify and revise your plans and intervention in partnership with the service users.

    6.5   Any decision to cease intervention is based upon your evaluation and is taken in consultation with the service users.

    6.6   Your outcomes demonstrate the value and benefit of your input to the individual and/or community.

7. **You keep care records that are fit for purpose and process them according to legislation.**

    7.1   You provide a comprehensive, accurate and justifiable account of all that you plan or provide for service users.

    7.2   You record the evidence and rationale for all that you do.

    7.3   Your care records are written promptly, as soon as practically possible after the activity occurred.

7.4 You are aware of and meet all requirements in relation to record keeping, whether in legislation, guidance or policies.

7.5 You comply with any legal and professional requirements and local policies in relation to confidentiality, the sharing of information and service user access.

7.6 You keep your records securely, retain and dispose of them according to legal requirements and local policy.

> ➤ You are advised to read the College of Occupational Therapists' current guidance on *Record keeping* (COT 2010a) for further information. A third edition is due for publication in 2017.

8. **You seek to demonstrate and enhance the quality, value and effectiveness of the service/s that you provide.**

8.1 You collect and collate outcome data to evidence the effectiveness of your interventions.

8.2 You collect and collate outcome data to meet the requirements of commissioners/funders of services.

8.3 You seek to measure the impact of your input on the occupational performance, participation and wellbeing of service users.

8.4 Where possible you collect and use data to demonstrate the value for money of the service/s that you provide.

8.5 You use the information that you collect, with other national, local and professional resources, to improve the quality, value and effectiveness of the service/s that you provide.

9. **You are qualified by education, training and/or experience to practise capably and safely in your chosen role.**

9.1 You have sufficient knowledge and skills to make reliable professional judgements suitable to your level of responsibility.

9.2 You only work within your professional competence, seeking advice or referring to another professional when required.

9.3 You continually maintain your knowledge and skills in order to meet the needs of service users safely and effectively.

9.4 You maintain your awareness and skills in digital technology in order to meet the requirements of your role.

9.5 You participate in any statutory and mandatory training required for your work.

9.6 You seek out and engage with continuing professional development opportunities relevant to your learning and development needs, to encompass practice skills, research skills, teaching others and leadership.

9.7 You receive the equivalent of a minimum of one half day each month for agreed continuing professional development activity, scholarship and/or research (RCN et al 2007), over and above statutory and mandatory training.

9.8 As a practitioner, you receive regular professional supervision and appraisal, where you use critical reflection to review your practice.

> ➤ As part of your CPD, you are advised to read the College of Occupational Therapists' *Managing information: a 10-year strategic vision for occupational therapy informatics* (2014b) and the accompanying *Managing information: implementation plan 2015–2025* (COT 2015c).
>
> ➤ You are also advised to read the College's current guide on *Supervision* (COT 2015d) and the *College of Occupational Therapists code of continuing professional development* (COT 2015a, appendix 2) for further information.
>
> ➤ Further additional reading includes the College's *Entry level occupational therapy core knowledge and practice skills* (COT 2016) and the forthcoming publication (in development at the time of press, due late 2017) *The career development framework: guiding principles for occupational therapy* (COT in press).

10. You work collaboratively with your colleagues to maximise the outcomes of intervention.

10.1 You actively seek to build and sustain positive professional relationships.

10.2 You work and communicate with colleagues and representatives of other organisations to ensure the safety and wellbeing of service users.

10.3 You work with others within your area of expertise to promote knowledge, skills and good practice.

10.4 You refer to other colleagues or services where appropriate, utilising their skills to the benefit of the service user.

11. **Your communication style and manner is always professional.**

11.1 Your language and communication style demonstrates respect to those with whom you are working.

11.2 You always maintain professional communication towards your colleagues and/or service users.

11.3 You communicate with service users clearly, openly, sensitively and effectively.

11.4 Discussions related to service users are held in a way that maintains their dignity and privacy.

11.5 You confidently participate in formal and informal reporting.

11.6 You communicate effectively within your line management structure.

11.7 You document your comments where a written record is needed.

12. You support the training and development of colleagues and those you supervise.

12.1 You provide regular supervision and annual appraisals to those you line/professionally manage.

12.2 Where appropriate you provide regular practice education opportunities for occupational therapy students, in accordance with relevant standards.

12.3 You support the learning and development of colleagues from other professions, services and agencies in relation to occupational therapy.

13. You monitor, make best use of and sustain your personal and service resources.

13.1 You recognise the limits of your own capacity and do not extend your workload or remit to the detriment of the quality or safety of your service.

13.2 You seek to work as effectively and efficiently as possible to make best use of environmental, physical, financial, human and personal resources.

13.3 You ensure that your service meets the ongoing needs of the service user population.

13.4 As a practitioner you report and document where resource and service deficiencies may endanger the health and safety of service users, carers, yourself and your colleagues.

13.5 As a manager, clinical or professional leader, you act on any reports concerning resources and service deficiencies.

14. **You take reasonable care of your own health and safety and that of others who may be affected by what you do, or do not do.**

14.1 You abide by national and local health and safety regulations, policies and procedures.

14.2 You abide by national and local risk management regulations, policies and procedures.

14.3 You enable positive risks to be taken safely by service users, in cases where such risks are a necessary part of intervention.

14.4 You establish and maintain a safe practice environment, including when travelling or in the community.

14.5 You abide by legislation and guidance concerning moving and handling, while enabling service users to gain optimal occupational performance and autonomy in their lives.

14.6 You ensure that you, and those for whom you are responsible, are trained and competent in moving and handling techniques, including the selection and use of equipment.

> ➤ You are advised to read the College's current guidance on *Risk management* (COT 2010b) for further information. A new edition is due to be published in late 2017.

References

Bonnard M, Anaby D (2016) Enabling participation of students through school-based occupational therapy services: towards a broader scope of practice. *British Journal of Occupational Therapy, 79(3),*188–192. Available at: *http://bjo.sagepub.com/content/79/3/188.full.pdf+html*

Caparo Industries plc v Dickman [1990] 2 AC 605 (HL).

Christiansen CH, Townsend EA eds (2004) *Introduction to occupation: the art and science of living.* Upper Saddle River, NJ: Prentice Hall.

CIPD (Chartered Institute of Personnel and Development) (2016) *What is CPD?* London: CIPD. Available at: *https://www.cipd.co.uk/cpd/about.aspx*

College of Occupational Therapists (in press) *The career framework: guiding principles for occupational therapy.* London: COT.

College of Occupational Therapists (2016) *Entry level occupational therapy core knowledge and practice skills.* London: COT.

College of Occupational Therapists (2015a) *Code of ethics and professional conduct.* London: COT. Available at: *https://www.cot.co.uk/sites/default/files/publications/public/CODE-OF-ETHICS-2015.pdf*

College of Occupational Therapists (2015b) *Measuring outcomes.* (Research Briefing). London: COT. Available at: *https://www.cot.co.uk/briefings/measuring-outcomes-2015*

College of Occupational Therapists (2015c) *Managing information: implementation plan 2015–2025.* London: COT. Available at: *https://www.cot.co.uk/ publication/z-listing/managing-information- implementation-plan-2015-2025*

College of Occupational Therapists (2015d) *Supervision.* London: COT. Available at: *https://www.cot.co.uk/publication/z-listing/supervision*

College of Occupational Therapists (2014a) *College of Occupational Therapists' learning and development standards for pre-registration education.* London: COT.

College of Occupational Therapists (2014b) *Managing information: a 10-year strategic vision for occupational therapy informatics.* London: COT. Available at: *https://www.cot.co.uk/publication/ cot-publications/managing-information*

College of Occupational Therapists (2011) *Professional standards for occupational therapy practice.* London: COT.

College of Occupational Therapists (2010a) *Record keeping.* 2nd ed. London: COT. Available at: *https://www.cot.co.uk/publication/books-guidance/ record-keeping*

College of Occupational Therapists (2010b) *Risk management.* 2nd ed. London: COT. Available at: *https://www.cot.co.uk/publication/books-z-listing/risk- management*

Eriksson L, Welander J, Granlund M (2007) Participation in everyday school activities for children with and without disabilities. *Journal of Developmental and Physical Disabilities, 19(5),* 485–502.

European Network of Occupational Therapy in Higher Education Terminology Project Group (2004) *Occupational therapy terminology database.* Amsterdam: ENOTHE. Available at: *http://pedit.hio.no/~brian/enothe/terminology/*

Great Britain. Parliament (2005) *Mental Capacity Act 2005.* London: Stationery Office. Available at: *http://www.legislation.gov.uk/ukpga/2005/9/contents*

Great Britain. Parliament (1995) *Carers (Recognition & Services) Act 1995.* London: HMSO. Available at: http://www.legislation.gov.uk/ukpga/1995/12/contents

Harvey L (2014) *Analytic quality glossary.* [s.l.]: Quality Research International. Available at: *http://www.qualityresearchinternational.com/ glossary/#c*

Health and Care Professions Council (2016) *Standards of conduct, performance and ethics.* London: HCPC.

Health and Care Professions Council (2013) *Standards of proficiency: occupational therapists.* London: HCPC.

Health and Care Professions Council (2012) *Your guide to our standards for continuing professional development.* London: HCPC.

Hemmingsson H, Jonsson H (2005) An occupational perspective on the concept of participation in the international classification of functioning, disability and health – some critical remarks. *American Journal of Occupational Therapy, 59(5),* 569–576.

Hudson B (2010) *An asset-based approach to community building.* Surrey: Community Care. Available at: *http://www.communitycare.co.uk/2010/ 06/11/an-asset-based-approach-to-community-building/*

Jameton A, McGuire C (2002) Towards sustainable health-care services: principles, challenges, and a process. *International Journal of Sustainability in Higher Education, 3(2)*, 113–127.

O'Brian JC, Hussay SM, Sabonis-Chaffee B (2012) *Introduction to occupational therapy.* 4th ed. Missouri: Elsevier Mosby.

Royal College of Nursing, College of Occupational Therapists, Institute of Biomedical Science (2007) *A joint statement on continuing professional development for health and social care practitioners.* London: RCN.

UKCEN Clinical Ethics Network (2011) *Mental Capacity Act: determining best interests.* Warwick: UKCEN. Available at: *http://www.ukcen.net/index.php/ education_resources/mental_capacity/determining_ best_interests*

World Federation of Occupational Therapists (2016) Definition "occupation". Forrestfield, AU: WFOT. Available at: *http://www.wfot.org/AboutUs/ AboutOccupationalTherapy/DefinitionofOccupational Therapy.aspx*

World Federation of Occupational Therapists (2013) *Definitions of occupational therapy from member organisations.* Forrestfield, AU: WFOT. Available at: *http://www.wfot.org/ResourceCentre.aspx*

World Health Organisation (2002) *Towards a common language for functioning, disability and health ICF.* Geneva: WHO. Available at: *http://www.who.int/ classifications/icf/en/*

All websites accessed on 28.07.16.

Continued overleaf